Essential Oils

Essential Oils for Beginners Guide to Get Started with Aromatherapy and Essential Oils Recipes for Health and Healing

Second Edition

By
Jason Williams

© **Copyright 2017 by – Jason Williams – All rights reserved.**

This document is geared towards providing exact and reliable information in regards to the topic and issue covered. The publication is sold with the idea that the publisher is not required to render accounting, officially permitted, or otherwise, qualified services. If advice is necessary, legal or professional, a practiced individual in the profession should be ordered.

- From a Declaration of Principles which was accepted and approved equally by a Committee of the American Bar Association and a Committee of Publishers and Associations.

In no way is it legal to reproduce, duplicate, or transmit any part of this document in either electronic means or in printed format. Recording of this publication is strictly prohibited and any storage of this document is not allowed unless with written permission from the publisher. All rights reserved.

The information provided herein is stated to be truthful and consistent, in that any liability, in terms of inattention or otherwise, by any usage or abuse of any policies, processes, or directions contained within is the solitary and utter responsibility of the recipient reader. Under no circumstances will any legal responsibility or blame be held against the publisher for any reparation, damages, or monetary loss due to the information herein, either directly or indirectly.

Respective authors own all copyrights not held by the publisher.

The information herein is offered for informational purposes solely, and is universal as so. The presentation of the information is without contract or any type of guarantee assurance.

The trademarks that are used are without any consent, and the publication of the trademark is without permission or backing by the trademark owner. All trademarks and brands within this book are for clarifying purposes only and are the owned by the owners themselves, not affiliated with this document.

Table Of Contents

Introduction v

Chapter 1: Brief History of Aromatherapy 1

Chapter 2: Different Types of Aromatics 7

Chapter 3: Benefits of Essential Oils 17

Chapter 4: Methods for Using Oils 33

Chapter 5: Cautions and Safety 53

Chapter 6: Essential Oil Recipes 65

Conclusion 77

Introduction

I want to thank you and congratulate you for purchasing the book, *"Essentials Oils: Essential Oils for Beginners Guide to Get Started with Aromatherapy and Essential Oils Recipes for Health and Healing"*.

This book contains proven steps and strategies on how to take advantage of the therapeutic benefits of pure essential oils so you can heal yourself the natural way. You will find practical tips and recipes as well as safety guidelines so you can maximize the potential of any aromatic oil.

People have been practicing aromatherapy for thousands of years, but because of advances in medicine and drug manufacturing, the practice of average individuals using essential oils for improving health and wellness has been regarded as ineffective and having no basis in science. However, the work of modern researchers and scientists are still being influenced by what ancient civilizations already knew - the use of essential oils has positive effects on both the body and mind.

Thanks again for purchasing this book, I hope you enjoy it!

CHAPTER 1

Brief History of Aromatherapy

You may have heard the term "Aromatherapy" lately and probably wondered if it's a modern form of alternative medicine. Well, in truth, aromatherapy has been in practice since the ancient civilizations, but the actual term had not been coined until the early 20th Century. Aromatherapy started several thousand years back with the practice of extracting botanical oils for various healing and religious purification purposes.

Ancient Origins of Aromatherapy

The use of plant extracts and oils for medicinal use started approximately 3,500 years before Christ. Ancient civilizations across the globe have revered aromatic plants and have used them in healing both the body and the mind.

Ancient aromatherapy has been closely linked with medicine, mysticism, and religion. Most ancient people also used aromatic plants to help them seek mind-body balance.

Here's how aromatherapy started within the ancient civilizations.

- **Chinese Culture**

  Aromatherapy's roots are believed to have started in Ancient China. The oldest surviving medical book in China named "Yellow Emperor's Classic of Internal Medicine" contains valuable information about several plants and their medicinal uses. The book, which dates back to 2697 BC, is among the earliest known recordings of ancient people using plants for medicinal purposes.

The ancient Chinese extracted oils from various medicinal plants and burned them as a part of tribal religious worship. Burnt oils were also extensively used as herbal remedies for illnesses.

Herbal burnt oils were also incorporated by the Chinese during ancient massage and acupressure sessions.

Ancient Chinese people also believed that their moods can be improved by taking whiffs of burnt plant oils or by incorporating them in relaxing massage sessions, very similar to the beliefs that modern aromatherapy holds true today.

- **Egyptian Culture**

It had been widely known that Egyptian people were also pioneers in aromatherapy, alongside the Chinese.

Ancient Egyptians mainly used cedarwood, cinnamon, and myrrh plant oils for embalming their dead. They also used frankincense for preserving their dead during mummification.

Egyptians also discovered perfumes, and used these fragrant oils for calming sick people who were to undergo traditional healing sessions. Perfumes made from fragrant plant oils were also used by women in anointing their bodies after their baths.

Fragrant plant oils were also used in creating the Kyphi. This substance is used as temple incense and is also used for treating lung and liver illnesses. Kyphi includes some plants such as cardamom, juniper berries, cinnamon, and saffron in its list of ingredients.

- **Indian Culture**

Ancient Indian natives used Ayurveda/Ayurvedic medicine, one of the earliest forms of holistic mind-body healing systems. Ayurveda is based on the concept of recreating a sick person's body, mind, and spirit through the use of herbal remedies.

Sandalwood played an important role in ancient Ayurvedic medicine practice. Burnt sandalwood was used in driving away evil spirits during exorcism. The plant is also used to treat various kinds of wounds.

To this day, most Indians still believe and practice Ayurveda in several small forms, as an adjunct to modern medicine.

- **Greek Culture**

The ancient Greeks were the ones who expounded on the use of aromatherapy plant oils. Notable Greek medicine figures have used plant oils in a variety of healing procedures that they pioneered.

Hippocrates was the great Greek physician famous for his belief that the human body should be treated holistically as a single organism. He further advanced his studies to include herbal medicine, and studied over 200 plants and their medicinal benefits. He was the first physician to use plant oils in healing baths and soothing massages. He also discovered chamomile's ability to reduce fever.

The founder of botany also sprang forth from the ancient Greeks. Aristotle's student Theophrastus was regarded as the Father of Botany because of his extensive work on learning things about plants and how they affect the human emotions.

Dioscorides was another Greek physician who lived from 40-90 AD. He studied the medicinal properties of herbs while joining the Roman armies in their journeys to Italy, Germany, Spain, and Greece. He recorded all of his findings in a book called "De Materia Medica", also known as the "Herbarius". This book contained descriptions of over 100 different plants, including thyme, peppermint, myrrh, almonds, chamomile, ginger, cardamom, coriander, dill, poppy, sesame, and rhubarb.

Claudius Galen was the last Greek physician to use medicinal herbs and plant oils for healing. Galen worked under the Romans to treat wounded gladiators. He studied his gladiator patient's various wounds and came up with using herbs to treat them. He also created various formulations combining several plant oils to be used as remedies for illnesses. One particular formulation was a mixture of rose petals, olive oil, beeswax, and water, which served as the first cold cream for cosmetic use.

Greek mythology also showed how important plant oils were to the Greeks. Asclepius, the Greek god of prophecy and healing, was taught by his divine father Apollo the secrets of healing through herbs and medicinal plants.

Aromatherapy During the Middle Ages

After the important contributions of several ancient civilizations on aromatherapy, the science of medicinal plants and aromatic plant oils continued to flourish during the middle ages.

Distillation techniques were discovered during the Medieval Period, under the Roman Empire. Avicenna, a Persian physician, uncovered this technique and used it to process raw plant oil extracts. He specifically used steam distillation to extract rose essential oils. He used his newly-distilled plant oils for promoting general good health through various massaging techniques.

The popularity of aromatherapy somewhat declined during the Medieval Ages. Credits were given to Christian monks who continued to use herbal medicine and aromatic plants as traditional cures for illnesses.

Aromatherapy Beyond the Dark Ages

Using botanical essences as medicine piqued the interest of several scientists and physicians after the Dark Medieval years. Among them was Nicholas Culpepper, an English botanist who engaged in a deep study about the healing properties of various plants. He even published his botanical encyclopedia titled "Complete Herbal", and used his findings on herbal remedies in curing sick people of his time.

From there on, the studies carried out regarding plants and their health benefits never ceased. People became more interested in botanicals and aromatherapy more than ever, up to the present time.

Coining the Term "Aromatherapy"

Aromatherapy is the use of natural plant oils, or essential oils, to heal both the body and mind. The practice dates back to the ancient civilizations, but the term 'aromatherapy' was coined by René-Maurice Gattefossé in his 1937 book *Aromathérapie: Les Huiles Essentielles, Hormones Végétales*. He was a chemist working for his family's perfumery business in France. After discovering that lavender oil healed an accidental burn on his hand, he went on to discover the properties of other oils.

In his book, he also articulated that natural oils were vastly superior to synthetic oils in terms of healing. This echoed the discovery of Cuthbert Hall in 1904 who presented that pure eucalyptus oil was much more potent than its synthetic counterpart, eucalyptol. Later scientists sought to explore the specific medical disorders that the essential oils can treat.

The term 'aromatherapy' is a misnomer because it suggests that it is a form of therapy or healing done through smell. It can mislead people since they would think that only through smelling essential oils will they be healed from their illnesses.

However, the term generally pertains to healing using essential oils. Aside from their scent, which is in itself already healing, oils can also alter the body's chemistry by targeting other senses and bodily functions. Massage therapy is one way to introduce essential oils to the body through the skin. Therefore, it is not just the aroma, but the way the body interacts with the oils that lead to healing.

Today, modern aromatherapy strictly only uses essential oils externally. Placing aromatic plant oil concoctions on a person's external body is actually feasible enough to help it recover from various illnesses.

The potency of oils can lead to higher concentrations, having adverse effects on the body. So, essential oils are almost always prepared in a solution of other natural substances like carrier oils (e.g., castor oil, coconut oil, sunflower seed oil), balms (e.g., beeswax, shea butter, cocoa butter) or liquids (e.g., water, alcohol, witch hazel) before applying directly onto the skin.

Studies also show that some essential oils are more effective when inhaled rather than ingested. Chapter 5 has comprehensive safety guidelines when it comes to using essential oils.

CHAPTER 2

Different Types of Aromatics

Take a look at that bottle of aromatherapy essential oil you have with you. Can you recognize what are the plants it was taken from? And can you identify what primary source was used to create your aromatherapy oil?

Aromatic essential oils often come from one main source – botanical aromatic plants. The plant extracts form the central basis of the aromatherapy oils. But apart from that, there are other different types of aromatic essential oils that get their fragrance and healing properties from other sources.

Listed underneath are some of the different types and sources of aromatic essential oils:

Natural plants

Plants are the main sources of many aromatic oils. This is what gives them flavor and scent. Plants also keep these oils healthy and protect them from disease and pests.

Oils can be extracted from various plant parts, such as flowers, fruit juices, fruit peels, leaves, bark, root, wood and sap. Oils are extracted naturally by squeezing plant parts that contain abundant extracts. For instance, fresh citrus extracts are obtained by expressing the juice from the fruit and peels.

Chamomile, ylang ylang, rose, and jasmine store their essential oils in their flowers. These plants have their buds and petals crushed and squeezed to extract the oil. Cinnamon oil is extracted from the plant's bark, while cumin, dill, and cardamom are examples of plants where oil is extracted from their seeds.

However, not all plants contain essential oils. Scientists are still unclear about the reason for this, but it is known that they are important to the plant's life cycle.

One kind of tree can produce different types of oils like the orange tree where neroli oil comes from the flowers, orange oil comes from the bitter orange fruit peels, and petitgrain from the twigs and leaves. The methods of extraction vary but their origins can be traced back to ancient times.

Nowadays, plants bearing essential oils are cultivated in mass numbers to allow people to extract more oils for commercial and natural medicinal purposes.

Historical plants and oils

Oils have been used for healing since the time of the ancient civilizations. Plants are highly regarded and respected by the ancient people not only because of the food and shelter they provide, but most importantly because of their powerful healing extracts.

Plants were often regarded as a precious gift from the gods because they display life-sustaining properties. Ancient people extract plant oils and use them in various facets of everyday life.

There is an archaeological evidence that suggests that they were used for cosmetics, cooking and medicine, and many of these practices have sacred meanings attached to them. For the ancient people, plants are sacred things. Hence, they practiced several rituals with plant oils such as myrrh forming an important part of the celebrations. Until today, many religions still use some forms of aromatics in their rituals like frankincense in Roman Catholic services and burnt juniper in Tibetan worship.

Healing is the foremost reason why people took great interest in plant extracts. In the course of human history, people from different ancient civilizations had their own notable ways of using plant extracts to heal wounds, illnesses, and to drive away evil spirits. Several texts gleaned from various historic times bear witness to the importance of plant extracts in ancient medicine.

Old literature like the Rig Veda, precursor to later Hindu texts, mention hundreds of substances for use in healing such as cinnamon, sandalwood and myrrh. Chinese traditional medicine also utilized opium, camphor and ginger dating back to 2000 B.C. Egyptian culture is as well defined by oils with their use in the embalming process and for curing illnesses that were common to people back then.

Many of the oils known to the West today were first imported from the Asia continent including camphor from Borneo, rose from Syria and cinnamon from India. Along with this trade, knowledge of their healing properties was also shared to the rest of the world. The ancient Greeks and Romans were very interested in their use in perfumery and they created various fragrances for the body and household.

To this day, most countries in Asia and Europe find the importance of essential plant oils relevant in the modern world. They recognize the many advantages of aromatherapy with respect to helping sick people recover from illnesses. People note that the medicinal properties of plants that their ancestors were indeed effective. Hence, people of today preserved the learnings and teachings of their ancestors regarding aromatic plants. Aromatherapy was thus born, and is extensively used today either as a stand-alone natural therapy or as an adjunctive therapy alongside modern medicine.

Apart from medical uses, historic plant extracts were also used to create perfumes and other household items such as bath oils, soaps, and lotions. These items continue to help improve the health of people by preventing illness and promoting good health and hygiene.

Alchemy

Alchemy is a philosophical and scientific tradition borne out of man's earliest beliefs in human science. Its roots hail from the Hellenistic period of Egypt, and extends to the Roman Empire and finally, to medieval Europe.

Alchemy and aromatherapy are intricately woven together through the practices of extracting ancient plant oils. Distilling objects into its purest forms are ultimately thought as the best manifestations of divinity, and this alchemical principle became the basis for extracting plant oils. Ancient alchemists believed that turning plants into pure essential oils enable plants to pour out divine powers into human hands. That is why ancient alchemists channeled all their knowledge and skills to determine the best possible methods of extracting plant oils from various plant parts.

Alchemy became one of the sources of plant oils because modern oil distillation practices can be traced back to ancient Arab alchemists.

The ancient art of alchemy has origins in the practice of distillation. A 1975 expedition to the Indus Valley at the foot of the Himalayan mountains revealed that the distillation process known today was done by the Arabs in the preparation of aromatic oils four thousand years ago.

Arabs pioneered the process of steam distillation to extract the essential oils from various plant parts. Avicenna, a Persian thinker and physician, obtained rose essences through early methods of steam distillation. He even wrote one book solely dedicated to rose oil extracts.

Other notable Arab figures began expounding on various distillation practices. Among them was Al-Kindi, an Arab philosopher who described several kinds of essential oils in his book "The Book of Perfume Chemistry and Distillation". Jabir ibn Hayyan, another prominent natural philosopher hailing from the Umayyad Caliphate, wrote dedicated chapters on distillation processes in his book "Summa Perfectionism".

Arabian scents became popular in Europe throughout the Middle Ages. They were especially useful as protection from the plague and to mask the stench of the diseased. Because Asian gum trees were not yet being cultivated in Europe, the 14th to 16th century also saw the invention of many essential oils created from native plants like rosemary and lavender.

At the time, alchemy was more of a spiritual rather than a scientific pursuit. The ability to distill a substance to its purest form - perhaps gold - was the manifestation of the divine. However, the Scientific Revolution that occurred during the Renaissance propelled the practice towards a more academic discipline.

Scientific Creations

Not all plants have essential oils. And not all aromatic plants can be continuously cultivated for oil extraction purposes alone. Hence, present-day scientists created ways for essential oils to be replicated almost exactly as their original oil counterparts. Nowadays, essential oils can be obtained through various modern scientific methods.

Increased interest in the study of botanical plants and aromatherapy gradually hyped as the Middle Ages approached. It is during this period when the medicinal properties of aromatic plants took center stage.

The Middle Ages saw the coming of several kinds of diseases, such as pneumonia, leprosy, smallpox, St. Vitus' Dance, St. Anthony's Fire, scurvy, and dysentery. All these diseases plagued the entire European continent and were responsible for taking the lives of many people. The Black Plague of the 14th century also made health matters worse. No one knew what illness they were facing at that time. The deadly pandemic swept over 14th century Europe, killing millions of people in a span of five years.

All throughout these times, essential oils played an important role in trying to keep the people safe from all these fatal diseases. People started to burn pine and rosemary incense in their homes and on the streets.

They hoped these incenses will help protect them from the deadly Black Plague. Handkerchiefs were immersed in essential oils and were used to cover people's noses and mouths every time they go out of their homes.

During that time, it was believed that the deadly substances causing the Black Plague were carried through air contaminants, and the handkerchiefs laden with essential oils were thought to keep them safe from contracting the air contaminants causing the disease. Doctors would also wear beak-like masks filled with essential oils and plant extracts to keep them safe while treating their patients.

Pharmacists studied the healing effects of essential oils on various epidemics. In the early days of chemistry, they provided records of the properties of oils and combinations that are effective on various ailments. At the same time, perfumery developed into a separate specialty from apothecary. So, alchemy became chemistry, but was still guided by the alchemic principles of the connection of the body (biology) to the spirit (psychology).

During the 1700s, use of essential oil in medicine rose all the more. The European population rapidly increased in number, which triggered an increase in people without knowledge or access to facilities that can help them maintain sanitary and hygienic body conditions. During this period, doctors started to bring essential oils in their medical kits to help sanitize the people and to help promote good hygiene practices. Essential oils that they carried around included thyme, frankincense, juniper, sage, rose, rosemary, and lavender.

With the entry of the Modern Period came the significant changes in the way society viewed aromatic plants and essential oils. Scientists started to study the chemical composition of essential oils. They discovered specific properties of these oils that made them beneficial to the people. Examples of these properties include anti-bacterial, antiseptic, and anti-inflammatory effects.

Through the invention of scientific methods, chemists were able to isolate and name substances to identify them according to observable characteristics. This also paved the way for the creation of synthetic oils and modern drugs.

The use of plant extracts for medicinal purposes gradually declined since the advent of modern medicinal drugs and synthetically-produced plant essences. The demand for more pharmaceutical products pressed hard on the aromatherapy industry. It's because essential oils can become hard to find, and would need lots of plant stocks in order to ensure continuous supply.

So, by the 20th century, aromatherapy became discredited as the drug industry flourished. Essential oils became relegated to their use in food, perfume and cosmetics, and the knowledge of their use in healing by individuals was somewhat forgotten.

Many pharmaceutical companies started manufacturing synthetic, laboratory-made essential oils for commercial use. They do not manufacture them for healing purposes because synthetic oils do not carry the same healthful properties that their real oil counterparts have.

It is quite paradoxical that during the era when essential oils were deeply researched and made well-known, it is the same era when their most valuable importance in medicine has been overrun by a flourishing manufacturing society.

Natural Oils Versus Synthetic Oils

At this point, it would be important to reiterate the difference between using natural oils versus synthetic oils. Also called fragrance oils, the latter may smell like the oils that they are copying, but they contain none of the healing benefits. Synthetic fragrance oils, hence, cannot be used as replacements or alternatives to real, organic essential oils.

These oils are created in a lab, so they do not have the biological properties of real essential oils. Furthermore, synthetic oils contain compounds that are hazardous to health. They may be sold at much cheaper prices than natural oils, but they are unsuitable for the purposes outlined in this book.

As its name suggests, it would be best to use fragrance oils for creating fragrances and you can usually find them as ingredients in most commercial perfumes, shampoos, lotions, other bath products and cosmetics.

Synthetic fragrance oils are created to meet the demands of modern-day users. Present-day manufactured products often require large amounts of essential oil, which may be hard to meet if traditional ways of extracting oil will be done. Plus, it would be expensive to source several aromatic plants and extract their oils rather than have these oils be made synthetically.

The biggest downside of this, however, is that synthetic fragrance oils are not potent and lack the original composition of real essential oils. Thus, they don't contain healthful properties and are not really suited for therapeutic-grade purposes.

Characteristics of Good Natural Essential Oils

Good essential oils ideally display the following characteristics to be identified as truly genuine:

- **Certified Organically Grown**

    Organic essential oils are grown free from any fertilizers, pesticides, and insecticides. This ensures that the essential oils extracted from the plants are pure, safe, and chemical-free.

    When choosing natural oils, it is best to opt for certified organic oils. These are certified by a third party as coming from a company with good harvesting and extracting practices that are ethical and sustainable for the environment. Some farmers may not be able to cope with the high costs of certification, so there are non-certified organic oils in the market.

Organic oils were supposed to be grown without pesticides and other harmful chemicals. This is especially rampant in large scale industrial farms that produce oils without natural insecticidal properties like those from less hardy flowers and fruits.

- **Harvested from the Wilds**

Plants that naturally grow in the wild forests and other natural thriving places usually yield the most potent essential oils.

Ideally, essential oils must be extracted from plants growing in their most natural thriving places. But then, it would be quite impossible to keep these sources abundant for continued oil extraction. And genuine oils produced from these natural thriving areas would be way too expensive than others. Plantations are then utilized for more cost-effective means to produce natural plant oils.

But still, the best kind of oils are those that are wild harvested. These are of high quality and are the best in the world because they are harvested from sources naturally found in the wild, rather than from plants that are cultivated for the purpose of harvesting them.

For example, there are different types of lavender oils in the market, which are usually differentiated by their origin. Those sourced from lavender that grows wild in high altitudes tend to be more potent than those harvested from a lavender plantation. This fact can be proven by examining the genetic makeup of wild lavender. They have stronger immunity to disease and harsh climate making them better for therapeutic use.

Thus, the source of essential oils is very important whether they be for personal use or for healing others.

- **Highly Concentrated**

Genuine natural essential oils are packaged in highly concentrated amounts. A single drop of pure essential oil goes a long way in providing therapeutic care for a variety of ailments.

One good way to determine the oil's concentration is to determine if the oil is richly fragrant or not. Concentrated essential oils are highly fragrant straight from their bottles. You need not take a deep whiff of the oils; some potent oils could be highly toxic when deeply inhaled in its concentrated form. You simply need to examine it quickly; the potent fragrance of genuine essential oils naturally comes out even without opening their bottles.

Natural essential oils are also packaged as it is, without any carriers or water to dilute it. Generally, high-quality natural essential oils are more viscous than their synthetic counterparts. Be wary of products packaged as essential oils that carry a thinner consistency. Such products might be synthetic fragrance oils, or they could be counterfeit.

Even just one drop of concentrated essential oil is sufficient enough to produce healthy beneficial results. For instance, only a small amount of oil drops is mixed with a carrier oil diluent that could be used for a large portion of the body.

CHAPTER 3

Benefits of Essential Oils

Many essential oils today are being exploited for use in drugs and medicinal preparations. This is because they contain active compounds that have positive biological effects. Most ancient sources may refer to these with an air of mysticism or magic, but it is possible to understand them in a modern way.

Herbs that are said to be "a cure for a broken heart" can be taken to mean as falling within the category of antidepressants. Even in antiquity, specific problems are addressed by particular oils.

Indeed, essential oils have several proven benefits on various aspects of the human body. These benefits are listed in this chapter and will be explained in order of the body systems that the essential oils can reach. Specific essential oils that exhibit the benefits stated are also explained.

Digestion

Most oils are not to be taken orally and topical or other types of external application is recommended. (See Chapter 4 for a discussion on methods.) This does present limits to the efficacy of essential oils over herbal remedies that can be ingested. However, there is still evidence supporting their positive effect on digestive problem such as stomach pain, spasms, nausea, flatulent dyspepsia, liver issues, blockages in the gall bladder, jaundice, loss of appetite and other eating disorders.

Such essential oils include chamomile, orange, peppermint, cinnamon, lemon balm, ginger, garlic, rosemary, basil and angelica:

- Chamomile essential oil contains antioxidant and anti-inflammatory properties that help soothe a frazzled gut. It also contains an antispasmodic substance called anodyne, which can help alleviate gas formation and relax the stomach's muscles. Chamomile essential oil is also used to stop nausea and vomiting.

- Essential oils extracted from orange can help alleviate constipation. It also helps in easing stomach cramps. Orange oil may be ingested; it acts as a gentle diuretic which helps you prevent bloating by increasing the production of urine.

- Peppermint oil can be ingested orally as a dietary supplement. It often comes in enteric-coated capsules to help the oils get dissolved and absorbed within a person's intestines. Peppermint oil eases the symptoms of irritable bowel syndrome, heartburn, and indigestion.

- Cinnamon oil exhibits an amazing ability to balance a person's blood sugar levels. It curbs a person's appetite and prevents him from overeating, which in turn gives the stomach ample space to do its digestion duties properly. Cinnamon oil is also great for stomach ulcers; the compound named eugenol present in cinnamon oil reduces the pain associated with various ulcer symptoms. The oil can also be used to combat parasite growth in the entire gut.

- Lemon balm is an herb that's used to effective combat colic, intestinal gas, bloating, upset stomach, and vomiting. The soothing and calming effect of lemon balm also works wonders in halting pain associated with digestive ailments and menstrual cramps.

- Ginger oil is often hailed as a great digestive system saver. Ginger oils exhibit good gastro-protective properties. It's one of the most widely used natural remedies for nausea, vomiting, stomach spasms, colic, diarrhea, and stomach aches.

- Essential oils extracted from garlic can be beneficial to people on a cleansing diet. Adding some garlic oil to their daily food helps promote peristalsis – the natural movements of the intestines – and therefore, help in pushing out unwanted substances trapped inside the gut. Garlic oil may also function as a good diuretic and intestinal parasite buster.

- Rosemary essential oil is useful in relieving generalized upset stomach. It efficiently eliminates gas pain and helps in stopping indigestion. The oils may be deeply inhaled to produce a calming effect and soothe muscle spasms experienced by a person's upset stomach. Rosemary also contains camosic acid and rosmarinic acid, two powerful antioxidants that help protect the digestive system from harmful elements.

- Sweet Basil oil exhibits carminative properties. That means that the oil is useful in relieving flatulence and expelling excessive gas from the digestive tract. It also helps relieve pain from stomach cramps.

- The sweet and spicy aromatic Angelica essential oil offers soothing properties for the spasm-plagued stomach. It is also great for removing intestinal and stomach gas. The oil can also stimulate the secretion of digestive juices such as bile, helping to stimulate proper functioning of the digestive system as a whole.

Immune System

Essential oils are mostly antibacterial and can help treat and guard against illnesses. It is for this reason why they gained popularity throughout the plague-ridden Middle Ages as people noticed that those who regularly use essential oils appear to have higher resistance to disease and faster recovery time.

Antibacterial and antiviral oils include bergamot, camphor, rosemary, clove, basil, lavender and tea tree.

- Bergamot's essential oil is derived from its rind and gives off a citrusy blend. This sweet-smelling oil contains germ-inhibiting compounds that ward off infections and stop the growth of bacteria. The oil is a constant ingredient in many antibacterial soaps. Bergamot oil can be rubbed onto the skin near the throat, feet, or stomach. Inhaling the vapors and scents of bergamot oil by using an oil vaporizer is also beneficial for fighting off bacteria in the body.

- Camphor oil is a potent antimicrobial and disinfectant. It can be used for disinfection of drinking water. It helps heal many skin infections, and is also a mainstay ingredient in ointments, creams, and lotions for skin diseases. Disinfecting the body can be done by mixing drops of camphor oil in bathing water.

- The woodsy yet minty aromatic Rosemary oil carries numerous antioxidants that are good for general health and well-being. But apart from that, rosemary oil contains the chemical carnosol, responsible for the anti-inflammatory and antibacterial properties.

- The strong-tasting clove oil is best used for toothaches with bacterial causes. Clove oil contains the active ingredient eugenol that is responsible for its antibacterial properties. This essential oil has long been in use for toothache relief even before the advent of modern dentistry.

- Basil oil has natural antibacterial and antiviral properties. Oils acting as antivirals can be rare, so take hold of some basil oil for viral infections. Basil oil contains active phytochemicals, antioxidants, and germ-busting eugenol and methyl chavicol compounds. Basil oil makes for a great remedy for colds; simply diffuse some oil in your home or make a vapor rub by adding

- some eucalyptus oil to it. Basil can fight off bacteria inside your body and even in your surroundings.

- Lavender oil is useful in treating acne. Active ingredients found in the oil gently inhibit the bacteria causing the acne breakouts. The oil's antibacterial property destroys the bacteria found on the skin and regulates excessive sebum secretion.

- Tea Tree Oil exhibits antiseptic properties, making it an excellent choice for treating various kinds of wounds. Tea tree oil can kill bacteria that cause several infections of the skin, nails, mouth, and teeth. A study found under the Journal of Investigative Dermatology showed an amazing discovery – tea tree oil can help kill staphylococcal infections and MRSA-related bodily infestations.

For healing, to reduce fever and to detoxify, oils that you can use include thyme, hyssop, angelica, peppermint, sage, lemon and eucalyptus.

- Thyme oil fights several strains of Staphylococcus bacteria, including MRSA. That's why it is a good natural remedy for chills and fever induced by bacteria. Apply oil drops on the chest, back, feet, and throat to gently soothe chills and fever.

- Hyssop oil is a natural antiseptic. It has powerful compounds that work against Staphylococcus aureus and Staphylococcus pyogenes, bacteria that may cause fever in humans. Reduce fever by massaging the soles of your feet with a concoction made from two drops of hyssop oil mixed with 1 mL of coconut oil.

- Angelica oil helps reduce fever by inducing diaphoresis. Perspiration carries unwanted toxins and waste products that can help clear up a fever faster. Angelica oil is also a diuretic, inducing urine flow to help lower fever.

- The cooling effects of peppermint oil are beneficial to someone suffering from fever and chills. Rubbing the oil on the neck and the soles of the feet does the trick.

- Sage essential oil's camphene and camphor compounds give it powerful antimicrobial and anti-inflammatory properties. The oil helps reduce inflammation, fight bacterial infections, and thus lower fever.

- Lemon oil can have powerful cooling properties that aids in lowering fever. Mix one drop of lemon oil to some peppermint oil and rub on the soles of your feet to reduce fever and fight off the infections causing it.

- Eucalyptus oil contains a compound called eucalyptol, famous for its fever-soothing properties. It gives the oil antiseptic properties as well. Combine eucalyptus oil with some peppermint oil and spray on your body to cool you down and lower your high body temperature.

Respiratory System

Inhaling essential oils has direct positive effect on nose, lung and throat problems. So, they can soothe the symptoms of many respiratory ailments along with curing them.

For coughs, the best oils to use include pine, thyme, eucalyptus, fennel, sandalwood and myrrh.

- Pine oil exhibits expectorant properties. It helps mobilize mucus secretions in the lungs and aids in safely expelling them, relieving you from sticky and hard-to-expel cough.

- Thyme oil is an approved natural remedy for upper respiratory tract infection, whooping cough, and bronchitis management in Germany. Thyme oil acts as a mucus expectorant, clearing your lungs of mucus secretions.

Essential Oils

- Eucalyptus oil acts as a decongestant. It clears up clogged airway passages and soothes irritated nasal passages with its cooling effect. Eucalyptus oil is often used in treating cough, colds, sinusitis, and nasal congestion. Inhaling its vapors or massaging drops of the oil on the chest provides relief from congestion.

- Fennel oil relaxes spastic nasal airway passages. It is used to treat respiratory problems with chronic coughing spiels.

- Sandalwood oil exhibits antiviral properties, making it an effective remedy for upper respiratory tract infections that are viral in nature. It also works as an expectorant, relaxing the airway passages while aiding in expelling hard to remove mucus from the lungs. Inhaling a few sandalwood drops placed on a tissue or handkerchief can provide cough relief.

- Myrrh oil benefits persons suffering from sticky mucus secretions and persistent cough. It has expectorant properties, reducing the amount of phlegm in the respiratory tracts and in the lungs. It also aids in decongesting the nasal airways.

For asthma, the oils include hyssop, bergamot, cajeput and cypress.

- Inhaling hyssop oil helps relieve airway spasms experienced by asthmatic people. It also calms anxiety that asthmatic people may feel during asthmatic attacks.

- Bergamot oil steam can be of great help to asthmatic people. It reduces cough and expels mucus secretions. The ethyl acetate compounds from bergamot oil can also reduce inflammation in the bronchial area.

- Cajeput oil loosens phlegm and helps it be expelled easily. Inhaling the vapors may aid in relieving congested airways. It's also an antispasmodic, aiding in healing spasms caused by asthma attacks. First-time cajeput oil users must take caution, though, because the oil is so potent it could lead to allergic reactions if not used properly.

- Cypress essential oil is an excellent antispasmodic agent that effectively treats asthma, bronchitis, and various symptoms related to it. The oil can clear congested air passages and relieve spastic episodes.

For flu and colds, oils include thyme, tea tree, borneol and sage.

- Thyme oil's antibacterial properties make it an excellent natural remedy for flu and colds. Inhaling its vapors or adding a few drops to your bath can yield good flu-busting results.

- Tea Tree oil contains calming compounds that help ease irritating symptoms of the common cold. It's also antibacterial, antiviral, and antiseptic, driving out harmful elements causing the colds and flu. Like thyme, it is best used in baths to provide natural comfort and relief from flu and cold symptoms.

- Borneol is actually a potent compound classified under terpene alcohols. It is mostly found in rosemary oil. It can also be found in the Chines herb called Bing Pian. It has antibacterial and anti-inflammatory properties that aid in reducing the symptoms of influenza. It also has sedative properties that calm the sick person.

- Sage oil has valuable antioxidant properties, which helps in the recovery and protection of persons suffering from flu, cough, and colds. It also soothes spasms caused by prolonged coughing.

Stimulants

There are oils with sedating or stimulating effects that positively affect the nervous system. They work effectively in balancing the systems of the body. They can also positively affect a person's mood.

For the overall health of the nervous system, nervines include clary sage, juniper and marjoram.

- Clary sage is a perennial plant with oils extracted from the entire herb. This essential oil protects the nervous system and has calming and mild sedative effects.

- Juniper berry oil has abundant amounts of polyphenol antioxidants and flavonoids. These substances help protect the body's cells from damage. The oil appears to help in boosting the nervous system's overall well-being. Inhaling the vapors from juniper berry oil triggers relaxation and helps the brain calm down.

- Marjoram is an herb closely related to the oregano. Essential oil of marjoram can be diffused and inhaled to bring about a calm sensation that soothes the entire nervous system.

Sedatives for easing stress include lavender, lemon, valerian, sweet marjoram, chamomile, sandalwood and bergamot.

- Lavender essential oil bears a classic yet refreshing scent that's truly calming and stress-busting. Lavender oil is actually used as a natural remedy for various neurological ailments such as anxiety, depression, migraines, and chronic stress.

- Sweet Marjoram oil blends well with lavender and other relaxing essential oils. Together, these oils help beat stress and anxiety.

- Lemon oil is great for alleviating stress because of its refreshing citrusy scent. Diffusing lemon oil brings about a cheery and bright atmosphere to a room. The oil is a great pick-me-up remedy that can quickly counter mental exhaustion, anxiety, nervousness, dizziness, and mental tension.

- Valerian essential oil is derived from a perennial flower growing natively in parts of Asia and Europe. This oil has been proven effective in improving mood, alleviating stress, decreasing anxiety, and creating healthy sleep patterns. Improved sleep quality ultimately leads to a great reduction of stress, leading to a healthier mindset and mood.

- Chamomile oil has a gentle scent that soothes the senses once inhaled. It acts as a mild sedative, triggering a calm sensation that helps fight off stressful feelings. It also helps alleviate feelings of depression, hopelessness, and anxiety.

- Sandalwood oil was often included in ancient spiritual rituals because it promotes mental clarity. Nowadays, its valuable calming properties are still being used to calm frazzled nerves, halt stress, and provide a calm and relaxing atmosphere.

- Bergamot oil's citrusy scent busts stress and invokes an uplifted mood. It's a popular natural antidepressant and nervous system relaxant. Bergamot oil can stimulate the production and release of hormones called serotonin and dopamine. These hormones, in turn, facilitate relaxation and mild sedation.

Stimulants to combat fatigue include jasmine, peppermint, ylang ylang, basil, rosemary and angelica.

- Applying a few drops of jasmine oil to your skin can instantly uplift your mood and invigorate your senses. Diffusing this essential oil into the air yields the same benefits. Jasmine oil has a strong yet pleasant floral scent that helps improve mood, combat stress, fight fatigue, and eliminate sluggishness.

- Bring back your energy by using peppermint essential oil. This minty essential oil can stabilize mood, eliminate stress, and bring back vim and vigor for people with chronic fatigue. Apply it topically, diffuse it into the air, or inhale the vapors to achieve that energetic feeling.

- Ylang Ylang essential oil is also a widely known natural remedy for long-term fatigue and stress. This sweet Asian native oil displays mildly sedative effects that calms anxious persons. It can also lift up the moods of depressed and stressed people. Diffuse the oil or massage it on skin to enjoy its beneficial properties.

- Basil essential oil is a natural stimulant that helps combat chronic fatigue and brings back alertness and energy. Dab drops of this oil on your wrists, back, and chest to instantly hype your energy levels. Basil oil can also be massaged to the forehead to boost energy and lift up your spirits. You can also diffuse it or safely inhale the scents directly from its bottle.

- Rosemary plant oils melt down exhaustion through its active oxide component called 1.8 Cineole. This compound facilitates blood flow within the brain area, thereby leading to a reduction of fatigue and restoration of brain energy. Simply add one drop of pure rosemary oil to a cotton ball and inhale it once, one nostril at a time. You can also add it to your bath for a more calming experience.

- Recharge your stamina by using angelica essential oils. It provides an invigorating feeling every time it is inhaled or diffused into the air. The earthy and musky aroma of this essential oil enhances feelings of calmness and positivity.

Skin

Most essential oils typically benefit the skin in so many ways. Perhaps no essential oil will miss out on giving the skin a much-needed relief from various skin ailments.

Problems within the body often manifest as skin issues. This could be caused by an imbalance of hormones, toxin buildup and other failures in the systems of the body. Thus, the use of essential oils in skin care is widespread and varied.

Here are the various uses of essential oils for the skin. Examples of essential oils are included for each medicinal use explained below.

- **Antibacterial Skin Cleanser**

    Several essential oils contain antiseptic properties that help shield damaged skin from further infection. These oils also carry cleansing properties and can be used to decrease the number of bacteria thriving on wounded skin.

    For use as antiseptics to clean wounds and cuts, the oils that you can use include tea tree, juniper, cypress, lemongrass, lavender and sage.

    o   Tea Tree oil – The oil's powerful antibacterial and antiseptic properties are excellent in treating several skin conditions such as acne, psoriasis, boils arising from Staphylococcal bacteria, sunburn, sores, and insect bites.

    o   Juniper berry oil – Juniper oil exhibits good antibacterial properties. It has over 80 active compounds, including pinene, germacrene, and mycrene. The oil can help heal acne, reduce facial blemishes, decrease the appearance of stretch marks, and inhibit fungal growth in the feet. Juniper's sweet aroma can also help stop foot odors.

    o   Cypress oil – Camphene is the active antibacterial compound found in cypress oil. It inhibits the growth of bacteria and clears up any remaining bacteria that's currently thriving on the skin, preventing skin infections for both damaged and healthy skin. This essential oil is an excellent remedy for quickly healing external wounds like cuts, sores, pimples, and other skin eruptions.

    o   Lemongrass oil – The citrusy lemongrass oil is known to contain several antioxidants that can give skin a healthy glow. It also contains antibacterial properties that make it an effective skin cleanser. Lemongrass oil is an excellent natural toner and skin strengthener, and is great for keeping your skin healthily nourished.

o   Lavender oil – The relaxing lavender oil contains germ-fighting properties that make it a good choice for healing several skin ailments naturally. The oil can help hasten the skin's recovery from small cuts, scrapes, sunburn, age spots, and dry skin. Mix lavender oil with coconut or aloe oil for better skin care results.

o   Sage oil – Sage oil contains a number of natural compounds like pinenes and camphene, giving it antibacterial and antifungal properties. The oil is effective in treating skin conditions such as minor cuts, wounds, dermatitis, and fungal infections of the feet.

- **Natural Bug and Insect Repellent**

Essential oils can be used to ward off pesky insects such as mosquitoes, flies, and ants. Different insect-fighting oils contain various compounds that give them their mild yet effective insecticidal properties.

Bug repellents made from essential oils are generally safe and non-toxic than commercially-produced insecticides. There's less chemical residue that will be left on your body and on your surroundings when you use natural essential oils for repelling bugs.

Mild insecticides to fight off insects and bugs that bite and spread disease include the following: cedar wood, clove, camphor, citronella, eucalyptus, garlic, spike lavender, and geranium.

- Cedar wood oil – This oil's warm, wood-like aroma is actually toxic to insects. Cedar oil helps get rid of ticks, fleas, bed bugs, mites, and mosquitoes.

- Clove oil – The active ingredient Eugenol is responsible for its insect-killing properties. Use this oil to repel flies, moths, and ants.

- Camphor, Citronella, Eucalyptus, Garlic- These four essential oils are widely known as natural mosquito repellents. They are often found as ingredients in many mosquito repellent lotions.

  Camphor oil is one of the most potent natural mosquito repellents. It purifies the air while keeping mosquitoes at bay. Rubbing camphor on the skin also relieves the irritating itch brought about by mosquito bites.

  Citronella oil emits a natural scent that mosquitoes cannot stand. Citronella oil is often found in natural candles that are burned to prevent mosquitoes from infesting an area.

  Eucalyptus oil, like citronella, gives off a scent that makes mosquitoes confused and unable to reach their human hosts. The oil is often sprayed or rubbed on the skin. Eucalyptus oil also doubles as a good skin antiseptic for those already infested with mosquito bites.

  Essential oils extracted from garlic helps in repelling mosquitoes. Allicin is a compound found in garlic extracts, and is widely believed to cause their mild insecticide properties. Garlic oil's strong and pungent smell deters mosquitoes' sense of smell, disabling them from finding human prey to bite.

Essential Oils

o Spike Lavender oil – The insect-repelling power of spike lavender oil has been widely known even during the older times. People once used it to prevent moths from living in their linens and clothing. Nowadays, spike lavender oil can effectively repel black beetles, black flies, white flies, fleas, and mosquitoes.

Mix spike lavender oil with either eucalyptus or grapefruit oil and apply it to the skin to act as a natural insect repellent. Not only does it repel insects, it also helps heal skin that has been infested with insect bites.

- **Antifungal**

    Fungi is often hard to remove from infected skin, because its spores have the ability to live in the host's skin for months and years. Conventional antifungal drugs today can help kill fungal spores to eliminate the infection altogether. You have to keep on taking these medicines for years because even if the fungi are already visibly gone, spores could still remain and re-activate the fungal infection once your immune system becomes weakened.

    However, these drugs are often too expensive and can cost you several bucks because you have to continuously purchase them until your fungal infection completely disappears.

    That's where antifungal essential oils enter. Not only are these oils natural and synthetic chemical-free, they're also very effective in treating one-time and recurrent fungal skin infections. They're also more cost-effective than the conventional antifungal medicines in the pharmacy market today.

    Anti-fungal oils for ringworm or athlete's foot include: myrrh, patchouli and sweet marjoram.

- Myrrh essential oil is a good fungicide that can help eradicate skin fungal infections. Active compounds found in myrrh oil include sesquiterpenes and terpenoids. Myrrh oil is widely used to treat ringworm and athlete's foot. It can be applied topically by placing a few drops of the oil to a clean towel, then dabbing it on the affected skin.

- Patchouli is a bushy tropical plant hailing from Asia. Its essential oil comes from its dried leaves. Patchouli essential oil is used to heal athlete's foot and prevent foul-smelling odors caused by fungal infections.

- Sweet Marjoram oil exhibits more potent antifungal properties, compared to its close cousin oregano.

  A study conducted in 2000 and published in ACS Publications, Journal of Agricultural and Food Chemistry found the effectiveness of marjoram oil in inhibiting the growth of Penicillium digitatum, fungi specie causing green molds.

  Applying marjoram oil topically on the fungi-infested area yields the best results for treating fungal infections.

CHAPTER 4

Methods for Using Oils

So, you've already chosen an essential oil to use for healing your body from its various ailments. How will you apply that oil to your body?

You don't just go ahead and inhale or rub raw essential oils on your body. Essential oils have different entry modes, and it largely depends on what kind of oil it is and what particular benefit you want to get from it.

There are many methods that will allow your body to absorb essential oils effectively. They vary according to practicality and convenience, but what is most important is to choose a method that you simply prefer and you are comfortable with. A method may also be best suited for your purposes, so choose what you think will benefit you better.

There are six possible modes of essential oil administration in aromatherapy. These include inhalation, diffusers use, steaming, bathing, massage, and warm compress. Each method will be tackled in detail in this chapter.

Inhalation

Inhalation is one of the best and simplest methods to use essential oils. It's the approved method to treat several respiratory conditions, because the oil particles will obvious pass through the nasal passages and soothe them as they enter. And if your general health issue doesn't involve skin ailments involving topical remedies, then inhalation is your go-to method.

How Does Essential Oil Inhalation Work?

Open up a bottle of essential oil and gently take whiffs of the scent emanating from the oil itself. You'll likely feel a difference in your body and mind after a short while of doing so. But how did that happen? Here's a condensed scientific explanation:

Your nasal airways consist of the trachea, which branches out into bronchi. The bronchi further bifurcate into smaller and finer bronchioles. These bronchioles end in microscopic, air-filled sacs in the lungs called alveoli. It is in the alveoli where gas exchange and oxygen transport to the blood happens.

Upon inhaling the aroma of essential oils, the inhaled gaseous essences pass from the nose all the way down to the trachea up to the bronchi. The oil's gaseous particles disintegrate and pass through the small bronchioles, all the way down to the microscopic air sacs or alveoli. The tiny molecules coming from the inhaled oils then combine with oxygen and bind with fresh blood, ready to be distributed to the rest of the body.

That is how the nutrients from inhaled essential oils reach their targeted body parts internally. This whole process happens quickly, explaining why you experience instant feel-good bursts upon inhaling scents from aromatic oils.

Is Inhalation Safe?

Inhaling essential oils is generally a safe practice. There are certain oils that can be safely inhaled, and there are some that should be used in other methods and not for inhaling.

Direct inhaling of essential oils from their bottles is generally safe. But some essential oils approved for inhalation may require different diluted concentrations before use. Too much potency of a strong essential oil might do more harm than good if inhaled, so be sure to identify if your desired oil needs dilution. Follow the proper concentration in diluting with the proper carrier oils before inhaling them.

The following are examples of essential oils that can be safely used for direct inhalation:

- Chamomile
- Cinnamon Bark
- Citrus oils (Orange, Angelica, Bergamot, Lime, Grapefruit)
- Clove
- Frankincense
- Lavender
- Oregano
- Thyme
- Ylang Ylang

It is also important to note that high-quality, therapeutic-grade essential oils must be the only ones used for therapeutic inhalation. Synthetic fragrance oils may deliver similar scents, but they lack the healing properties of natural essential oils.

How to Do Inhalation Properly?

There are actually lots of ways to inhale essential oils. Choose one method that you're comfortable with. Stick to a method that brings you the calmest state and gives you the most health benefits.

Inhalation is actually the simplest method that you can do. Just open a bottle of essential oil and deeply inhale the scent to give you that extra boost of energy. This is perfect when you are feeling nauseous or you have a headache. Some oils can also help keep you awake or increase concentration, which is perfect for students who are studying or graveyard shift workers. It would also be good to pass an open bottle of essential oil under the nostrils of someone who has fainted or passed out. Doing so will wake them up and make them feel better.

When traveling, you can bring along small vials of essential oils instead of taking along their original bottles. This will also help preserve the potency of the oil because you are not frequently exposing it to air and light. (For more information on proper storage of essential oils, see Chapter 5.)

As an alternative, you can put a couple drops of diluted essential oil onto your palm, rub your hands together and cup them over your nose. Breathe deeply. Make sure that the essential oil was already mixed with a base or a carrier oil as undiluted essential oil could irritate the skin or be too strong to inhale. (Carrier oils will also be discussed in Chapter 5.)

If you do not want to use carrier oils, you can just put a couple drops of the essential oil straight on a cotton ball. Hold the cotton in your palm and cup over your nose.

Another good idea is to put a few drops of essential oils on your pillows. Three to five drops of essential oils are enough to give you that mild aroma you can inhale the entire night. This method is especially useful for people having a hard time sleeping and for those suffering from anxiety.

Diffusers

Diffusing oils with the help of various aromatherapy diffusers is another popular method of using aromatic oils. Diffused oils permeate every nook and cranny of your room, allowing you to inhale the aromatic particles for a longer period.

Aromatherapy Diffusers Defined

The device used in this method of essential oil use is called an aromatherapy diffuser.

An aromatherapy diffuser is a device that disperses an essential oil around a particular area. It works through the principle of diffusion – that is, the liquid particles of the oil move to a gaseous form and are allowed to spread over an entire area.

Aromatherapy diffusers come in different shapes and sizes. There are ones that are perfect for home or office use, as well as small ones that you can plug into your car or even in your computer's USB port.

Two most commonly used diffuser types include the following:

- **Cold-Air Diffuser**

Most diffusers now are powered with electricity and they work by vibrating the water molecules of the water and essential oil solution you pour into them. This type is called a cold-air diffuser.

Cold-air diffusers are also known as nebulizing diffusers. They are the gold standard when it comes to effective therapeutic use of essential oils. It's because these diffusers turn the essential oil's liquid matter into gaseous droplet particles without the use of heat.

You see, heat could possibly damage the original molecular structure of an essential oil. Using cold-air diffusers ensures that your essential oil's most therapeutic particles remain intact and floating around in the air for a longer period of time.

But be wary and careful in buying a cold-air diffuser. There are also cold-air diffusers marketed as humidifiers or air purifiers. Though they may seem similar, these products are usually not designed for essential oils. In fact, essential oils may even damage the units. These use fragrance oils or other special aromatics that work better.

Small downsides of using a cold-air diffuser include the use of electricity and the noise that can emanate from the motors of the diffuser. The noise might not be helpful for people who want a calming atmosphere to go with their essential oil diffusion. But modernity paves the way for the creation of more silent cold-air diffusers.

- **Warm Diffusers**

Another type of diffuser is the warm diffuser. These diffusers are sometimes bowls suspended over a tea candle. You light the candle so that the flame will warm up the essential oil mixture in the bowl. These can get too hot and boil the mixture. That is not ideal, because a slow warming of the mixture is better for the oils. There are also electric warm diffusers that you can plug into an electric source. These are not only safer but the temperature is much more controlled.

Warm diffusers can be classified as an evaporative oil diffuser. As the essential oil is slowly heated by the warm diffuser, its gaseous particles are released into the air through evaporation.

Heat may potentially lessen the amount of beneficial oil molecules in the air. But it does not completely destroy the essential oil's effectiveness. Some oil molecules actually remain intact; it's just that the potency of the essential oil might get a bit lessened. Warm diffusers are still fine to use because it still disperses air molecules coming from the warmed essential oils. You still get beneficial effects, but not as pronounced as when using a cold-air diffuser.

Warm diffusers also add up to the aesthetic value of your room. Various designs of bowls hanging over small candles can add flair to your room, creating a zen-like atmosphere while can actually help calm you down. Warm diffusers are also much quieter than cold-air diffusers.

For both cold-air and warm diffusers, the essential oils must be mixed with water first because pure essential oils are volatile and most of its components will evaporate instantly and will not diffuse properly in the air.

Is Diffusing Safe?

Diffusing oils is one of the safest ways to use aromatic oils. It's actually beneficial for people suffering from various respiratory conditions.

The benefits you get from diffusing are actually better than if you just inhale the essential oils for a short period of time. It's because the molecules coming from the aromatic oils are present in the air in droplet form for a longer period of time. You're able to get continuous oil particles as long as you stay in the room where the oils are being diffused. Thus, the health benefits you get from diffusing aromatic oils become more pronounced and continuous.

Who Should Use Diffusers?

People generally suffering from any respiratory ailment will greatly benefit from using aromatherapy diffusers. But more specifically, diffusers are good to use when you are suffering from sinus allergies or colds as they open up blockages in the nose and throat. Mint oils like eucalyptus, peppermint and spearmint (or even a combination of all of them) will be great for that purpose.

Diffusing oils would also be a good idea for people who want to create a peaceful and calming environment. This is useful for people suffering high levels of stress, anxiety, depression, and powerlessness. Staying in a room filled with aroma from the diffused essential oils will surely help uplift their spirits and improve their mood.

Steaming

Steam Inhalation is another method of using essential oils. It's a simple yet effective way of gaining relief from respiratory conditions, especially those that congest the nasal passages.

How Is Steaming Done?

Steaming is relatively easy. In a pot of boiling water, add a few drops of essential oil. Hover your face over the water and cover your head with a towel so that the steam does not escape and is allowed to circulate inside the towel. Remember to close your eyes and just relax. You can do this until it is still comfortable for you or once the water has cooled down enough.

Take deep breaths and inhale the steam deeply in order to feel the essential oil's effects. You should feel relief from congestion and an overall improved mood while the steaming process in ongoing.

Benefits of Steam Inhalation

The benefits of this practice include opening clogged sinuses, improving circulation, curing headaches and cleansing the pores of the skin.

- Steaming is especially useful for treating clogged airway passages. Essential oil drops are mixed with boiling water to create a relaxing steam that you can deeply inhale. As the medicated steam passes through the nasal sinuses and other airway parts, they dilate and widen. This allows nasal secretions to freely pass through, enabling the sick person to expectorate them better.

- Also, steaming is beneficial to soften hardened mucus secretions. Particles carrying expectorant properties from the essential oils are directly inhaled by the person through steaming. These particles go directly to the lungs through the nasal passages. The medicated particles act to soften thick, copious secretions, thereby making them easier to expel.

- Steaming can also improve blood circulation. The warm steam being inhaled goes to the lungs and is consequently picked up by the blood. The blood vessels expand to allow better blood flow. Along with oxygen, the blood also carries with it the healing properties of the particular essential oil being used.

- Inhaling medicated steam can also help cure headaches. The steam can have a relaxing effect that melts away headaches and provides a calm, relaxed feeling.

- Achieving beautiful skin is also possible through steaming. Improved blood circulation leads to an improved oxygen supply to the face, cleansing it from within. Large pores are also cleansed, minimized, and refreshed.

Is Steaming Safe?

Steam inhalation is a safe procedure as long as you've done it properly. You are dealing with heat and boiling water here, so necessary precautions to avoid accidental burns must be done.

Here are a few precautionary measures you must keep in mind while doing steam inhalation:

- Steam inhalation is good for respiratory ailments. But not all conditions may benefit from steam inhalation. If you suffer from hay fever, asthma, and allergic reactions, do not utilize steaming. The heat and steam coming from the boiling water might irritate your nasal passages and further constrict them, rendering the procedure ineffective and possibly even harmful to your condition.

- Steam inhalation is especially contraindicated in pregnant women suffering from high blood pressure. Excessive exposure to heat may trigger an increase in blood pressure and may potentially cut off blood circulation and oxygen supply to the baby.

- Children may use steam inhalation, provided that they are properly supervised. Do not allow prolonged exposure of a child to steam inhalation, as this increases the risk of burn injuries and scalding.

- Always be on the lookout for signs of possible adverse reactions such as difficulty of breathing, scalding, dehydration, and high blood pressure. Immediately stop the procedure once adverse reactions become evident.

- Be careful not to do this procedure too often as the heat may burst the tiny blood vessels in your face. Heat causes dilatation or widening of the small blood vessels. When you are exposed to excessive heat, your widened blood vessels might rupture.

- Also, do not use a pot over a heater or a self-heating pot because it will not cool down on its own and prolonged exposure to the heat is not advisable.

- If you are using an electric steam inhaler, fill it up with water only to an appropriate amount. Do not fully fill it up, because when you add drops of your essential oil, boiling water could splash out of the device.

- As a safety precaution, the steam inside the towel may also get too hot and the towel may touch the heater and catch fire. Be careful not to let the towel touch the boiling water or the heater.

Essential Oils for Steaming

Several essential oils can be used for steam inhalation. Oils that have proven benefits in treating nasal congestion and improving blood circulation are especially useful.

Here is a list of oils that can be beneficial in steam inhalation:

- Eucalyptus – This essential oil is an excellent natural treatment for cough and colds. It has antibacterial and decongestant properties.

- Peppermint – This oil contains powerful decongestant compounds. The minty nature of peppermint oil might be too strong, and care must be taken in order to avoid allergic reactions.

- Pine – Pine essential oil also exhibits decongestant properties, and is good for people who cannot take the strong scent of peppermint essential oil.

- Frankincense – This aromatic oil is a good choice for dry cough.

- Lavender – This relaxing essential oil also contains powerful antibacterial and decongestant properties.

- Tea Tree – Antiviral properties in tea tree oil make it an effective remedy for virus-induced upper respiratory tract infections.

You can add other ingredients into the water before boiling such as fruit peels or dried herbs to add more interesting aromas. See Chapter 6 for special essential oil recipes for facial steaming.

Bath

Essential oils can also be used in bathing. Warm baths infused with the goodness of essential oils can benefit your body in a myriad of ways.

How to Bathe with Essential Oils

Mix five to ten drops of your choice of essential oils in one half to one whole cup of emulsion like carrier oils, natural bath salts (e.g., sea salt, pink Himalayan), honey or milk. Then, draw your bath and add this mixture into the water. Soak in for as long as you please.

You may also dim the lights and play soft music in the background to enhance your relaxation and create a calm environment. You'll be able to further enjoy the benefits of your chosen essential oil by doing so.

Good Essential Oils for Bathing

There are several essential oils that are recommended for aromatic warm baths. These oils are as follows:

- Roman Chamomile
- Lavender
- Clary sage
- Frankincense
- Bergamot
- Citrus
- Myrrh
- Clove
- Vetiver

The next list features oils that must be used sparingly. The strong scents of these floral aromatic oils may become too overpowering when inhaled during a bath:

- Geranium
- Rose
- Ylang Ylang

Lastly, these oils should be minimally used because of their strong potency. They should be mixed with other oils to minimize the risks of irritation:

- Peppermint
- Spice oils such as cinnamon, ginger and black pepper

Benefits of Bathing with Essential Oils

Adding essential oils to your bath gives you lots of health benefits. You'd never think that soaking in a bath can be this good for your body and spirit.

The benefits of an aromatic bath include muscle relief (e.g., menstrual pains, cramps, fatigue), skin care, improved blood circulation and stress reduction.

- Soaking in a warm bath filled with essences from aromatic oils provides relief from muscular tension. The warmth of the water plus the relaxant properties of essential oils work together to calm stressed-out muscles, providing relief from cramping and fatigue.

- Women suffering from menstrual cramps and dysmenorrhea will also benefit from essential oils on a warm bath. Painful menstruation is often caused by sensitivity to the contractions of the uterine wall. The uterus is a muscle; hence, the same muscle-relaxing benefits of warm water bath and essential oils are also applicable to cramping uterine muscles.

- Bathing in aromatic oils is also a good way to care for your skin. Essential oils contain compounds that cleanse, disinfect, deodorize, and moisturize your skin.

- Essential oils added to a warm bath can also help enhance your blood's circulation. Soaking in the bath enables the active components of essential oils to penetrate the body and release their circulation-enhancing effects. Better circulation ultimately translates to better oxygenation of your body's tissues, recharging your energy and giving you fresh vitality.

- Stepping into an aromatic warm bath at the end of the day can ease all worries, stresses, and tension that you have experienced. Most essential oils have relaxant compounds that give off a calming vibe, which subsequently keeps your body and mind refreshed and relaxed. Bathing in aromatic oils and warm water also feels luxuriously good.

- Insomniacs can also benefit from a warm aromatic bath. The soothing and calming nature of baths plus the relaxing scents emanating from essential oils can help induce a restful sleep.

Considerations in Using Essential Oils in Warm Baths

You don't just add oil drops directly into your bath water. Here are some things you must know before you step into an aromatic warm bath.

- Oil and water does not mix together. Hence, you'll need to use an agent called emulsifier to blend your essential oils to your bath water. Emulsifiers enable better absorption of the essential oils on the water, and helps disperse the essences evenly. Use the proper emulsifier according to the oils you're about to use. Common emulsifying agents include the following:

    o   Polysorbates

    o   Natural bath gels

    o   Solubol

    o   Sulfonated castor oil

    o   Coconut emulsifiers

    o   Sesame oil

    o   Milk

- Ensure that the emulsifier and the essential oil are already thoroughly mixed before you add them to your bath water. Mix the concoction to your water just before you enter your bath tub.

- Do not add essential oils straight into the water without an emulsifier. The oils will stick to your skin instead of being gently absorbed by it. Be very careful because some oils are too potent to be directly applied to the skin. This could be irritating to the skin especially on sensitive areas.

- If irritation does occur, soothe the affected area with a mild oil (any carrier oil would do) or a gentle soap wash. Do not attempt to use plain water to wash it off as this will simply allow the skin to absorb oil better and will spread the oil on the skin faster.

Massage

Massage in itself is a great way to de-stress and re-energize the body and mind. Add essential oils to the mix, and you've got a great way to heal yourself from your ailments naturally.

Massage therapy is a directly topical way to apply essential oils on your body. This method is a wonderful way to use essential oils for healing and relaxation.

How to Use Essential Oils for Massage

As in the previously explained methods, essential oils are not to be applied directly to the skin. You need to dilute the oils first in carrier oils before using it on the skin. You can also concoct blends of essential oils to be used for any desired massage techniques.

You can use a variety of essential oil blends diluted in carrier oils to create a nice massage oil that is safe to use all over the body. A safe ratio is 15 drops of essential oil per ounce of carrier oil. For young children, the number of drop should be a third of the recommended drops for adults.

Milder, non-irritating essential oils like lavender, chamomile and clary sage can be used in higher concentrations of around 20 to 30 drops. Chapter 6 has fantastic massage oil recipes that you can try out for yourself.

Once you've blended your own massage oils, pour some in your hands and warm them up by rubbing your hands together. This is important so that you get a warm sensation as the oils are rubbed on your skin. You can then use the warmed oils to rub parts of your body that are afflicted by ailments.

Also, set the appropriate mood for a more relaxing massage. Light up some candles and play a relaxing tune in the background as you get yourself settled before the massage starts. A calm environment enhances the relaxing effects of your oil massage.

While being massaged, take deep breaths to inhale the scents of the oils being rubbed on your skin. The aroma of these oils can also have instant soothing and pacifying effects on your brain.

What Oils Can Be Used?

Popular essential oils that can be blended together to form massage concoctions include the following:

- Cedarwood
- Frankincense
- Coriander
- Lavender
- Cypress
- Sandalwood
- Peppermint
- Juniper
- Angelica
- Geranium

Benefits of Essential Oil Massage

Essential oil massage gives you a handful of health benefits:

- Essential oil massage is a luxurious way to treat yourself holistically. Massage coupled with essential oils is relaxing and stress-busting. It is a simple, fast yet effective way to ward off tension and stress. If you're feeling burned out, a quick massage can help you recover your energy.

- It stimulates blood flow in your skin and muscles, making them healthier. Essential oils are also easily absorbed by the skin, hence, the nutrients work their health benefits quickly while the massage is ongoing.

- Essential oil massage can ease cramps and pain associated with muscle tension. It's a good idea to have an essential oil massage if you're muscles have been feeling sore because of prolonged usage. It could be after standing around at work all day, or after you've just finished an intense workout routine.

- Massage can help heal wounds and skin conditions. Antibacterial and antiseptic properties penetrate the skin and release their beneficial compounds during a massage, helping heal the ailments and conditions afflicting your skin.

- Massage can also nourish your skin. Rubbing certain essential oils such as grapefruit and juniper oils helps cleanse and brighten dull and tired skin. Carrier oils used in diluting essential oils also provide moisture to the skin.

- Essential oil massage can help in meditation. Woodsy aromatic oils such as sandalwood and frankincense can be used to help you meditate and connect the body and the mind.

- It can also induce rest and sleep for people who have insomnia. The oil's fragrance can relax a person's senses, thereby helping them fall asleep faster. The quality of sleep is also better than those who do not use essential oils for overcoming insomnia.

Warm Compress

Essential oils may be incorporated to warm compresses to treat injuries in a natural way. It's simple to make and easy to use. They're used for bleeding control, alleviation of infection, and pain management.

Why Use Warm Compress?

Warm compress is an effective way to treat various wounds caused by trauma to the skin. The warm compress soaked with essential oils saturate the wound, providing quick antibacterial compounds to help heal said wounds faster.

Warm compresses also put pressure on wounds to aid in stopping continuous bleeding and to help in sealing the wound together.

What Oils Can Be Used?

Good essential oils to use for this purpose are tea tree and lavender oils that have antibacterial properties.

In addition to that, these oils can also be used to treat specific health conditions:

- For alleviating menstrual pain, you may use clary sage, lavender, chamomile, rosemary, peppermint, and rose oils.
- As a first-line natural treatment for boils and wounds with significant abscess, you may use eucalyptus, rose, bergamot, and tea tree oils.

- For general wound care, use lavender, frankincense, and tea tree oil.

- To help stop bleeding, you may use chamomile, lavender, geranium, tea tree, and rosemary.

How to Use Herbal Warm Compress?

For muscle aches and pains, wounds, cuts and bruising, compresses could be used. Just use a clean fabric like a towel and soak it in a cup of warm water mixed with around 10 drops of essential oil. Apply the warm compress on the affected area and leave until it has significantly cooled down. You may also reapply a second herbal warm compress as necessary.

Make sure that the water you use is not scalding hot as this may burn the skin or cause blisters. You can soak the towel in another warm mixture and reapply on the area if necessary.

CHAPTER 5

Cautions and Safety

Essential oils require special care and handling for its potency to last a long time. These oils are expensive because they were extracted from pure plant parts. Hence, it is rightfully important to be aware of how to properly store and use these oils. This is to avoid it being spoiled because of improper handling.

The use of aromatic plant oils also differs according to the purpose with which it will be used. Hence, there are certain precautionary measure you need to learn before using essential oils regularly. The safe use of essential oils lies in your knowledge of indications, contraindications, proper preparation techniques, and good safekeeping.

Storage and Care

Knowing how to properly store your essential oils is one key to preserve its freshness, potency, and healing properties. Here are some notes you must consider in proper storage and care of essential oils.

- Essential oils are highly volatile plant oils, so you must keep and store them properly so that they do not easily lose their potency. A liquid is volatile when it easily evaporates upon exposure to a certain temperature for a certain time period. When essential oils evaporate on their own because of mishandling or improper storage techniques, it gradually loses its potent medicinal properties and renders it less effective.

- However, real essential oils were distilled at temperatures of up to 140 degrees Fahrenheit, so leaving them out in a warm area will rarely alter their composition. They will return to their distilled state after cooling down. It is enough to store essential oils at room temperature.

- Keeping them in a cooler will not result in prolonged shelf life or better preservation. If they do get cold and turn waxy or solid, do not force them to liquefy by applying heat. Excessive heat can destroy particles that carry those important healing compounds within the oils. Allowing them to stand at room temperature is enough. Give the hardened oils ample time to return to their liquid state naturally.

- Applying direct heat is harmful to essential oils. As mentioned earlier, direct heat adversely affects an essential oil's healing properties, weakening its therapeutic benefits. So, even when using them in a heated diffuser, it is best to mix the oils with water first before lighting the candle or turning on the warmer. Temperatures of 300 degrees Fahrenheit and above will cause the more volatile compounds to disperse into the air faster, which minimizes the therapeutic effects.

- Have you ever noticed that essential oils come in dark bottles? There's sufficient reason behind it. Essential oils are best kept in amber-colored bottles or opaque heavy-duty containers to keep light out. Being exposed to light results in polymerization where the small molecules in the oil begin to separate from the bigger molecules. The small molecules often contain the most potent compounds that hold the oil's healing properties. Also, it is the small molecules that help in the absorption of the oil in the body.

- You may transfer essential oils from their original bottles to your chosen bottles, should you wish to bring essential oils any time you travel. But be sure to choose sturdy, dark-colored bottles that will last for a long time. Do not use low quality bottles to store essential oils as the cheap material of such bottles may affect the composition of the oils. Also, do not use bottles with rubber

Essential Oils

dropper caps. Many essential oils are sold in bottles with this type of lid; it's actually the most widely available bottle lids in our country.

And though the rubber dropper caps make usage easier, the rubber can turn into a gum and affect the oil inside in the long run. Instead, opt for simple vials with open tops, drip guards, pumps or droppers made of glass.

- Oxygen is essential oil's biggest enemy in keeping them fresh and potent. Air penetrating an opened bottle of essential oil enhances evaporation and decreases the oil's potency. It may also hasten your essential oil's decomposition. To address this problem, make sure that the bottles have lids or caps that you can securely fasten. This does not only help in preventing accidental spills or leaks, but this also helps in keeping the air out.

  Exposure to air is damaging to essential oils because its volatile components evaporate. Leaving the cap off for a while as you use the oil is fine, but do not leave it open for long periods of time. This is also why bottles with droppers (without rubber tops) are ideal for storing essential oils. They do not leave a lot of space for air to circulate in the bottle.

- Air also causes essential oils to go through the process of oxidation. Introducing oxygen molecules into the original components of the oil will change its particular structure and consequently, its healing effects.

- If possible, decant essential oils into smaller bottles and leave the rest in larger bottles. Use up the oils in the smaller bottles before refilling. This minimizes their exposure to light and air as most of the oils are left untouched, and they retain their original quality.

- If you've already used up half of the contents of a 2oz bottle (or any larger bottle of oil), pour the remaining half onto smaller bottles. Large bottles that are half-filled contain lots of airspace inside. In fact, the bottle contains half air and half oil already at that time. Transferring the contents to smaller bottles eliminates airspace and helps preserve the shelf life of the oils.

- Passing radiation through essential oils, as in the case of airport x-ray scanners, are believed to cause changes in the composition of the oil, albeit minimal. Electromagnetic energy does cause components in the oil to fragment—this is known by most as 'free radicals.' As we have been taught, free radicals are not good for the body as they cause cellular breakdown that lead to ageing, disease and other bodily issues.

  Oils that contain antioxidant properties may get oxidized when passing through enormously massive amounts of electromagnetic rays, damaging its antioxidant content and making it hard to fight off free radicals in the body.

- Nonetheless, the molecules in oil are small and only an insignificant amount would be hit by radiation and become fragmented. Also, essential oils are themselves antioxidants that fight against free radicals. In essence, oils are self-healing and will be able to recover on their own when minimally damaged. So, if your essential oils do have to go through a scanner, just allow for them to rest and repair for a while before using them.

- Essential oils are highly flammable liquids. When a certain oil reaches its maximum flashpoint threshold, it will ignite and burst into flames. Flashpoint is the term used to describe the highest possible temperature threshold required to ignite a flammable liquid. Hence, store your essential oils in a spot with normal room temperature. Avoid potentially fire-inducing areas such as wooden stove tops and kitchen ranges.

Safe Use of Carrier Liquids

Do you just open up a bottle of essential oil, place a few drops on your palm, and then rub them quickly on your ailing body parts? Not really, right? You see, there are pointers you need to consider before using essential oils. These pointers are designed to help you safely benefit from the oils and prevent adverse effects and potential injury as you use it.

One extremely important part of essential oil use entails the use of carrier liquids. Here are some reminders on the safe use of carriers for essential oils:

- Essential oils are dangerous to apply 'neat' or without a base. They are too concentrated and may irritate the skin. Make sure that you dilute your essential oils in carrier oil substances first. And be aware of the required number of oil drops needed to produce a certain oil-carrier concentration.

- Oil that has been mixed with the carrier diluent is a whole lot safer to use on the skin, rather than using the oils purely in itself.

  Also, it is easier to spread over large areas if they are mixed with other oils that are safer to use on the skin and are also cheaper to use in large amounts. And because essential oils have volatile components, carrier oils contain these active ingredients so that they do not dissipate into the air and are absorbed in the body. So, the chemical composition of the essential oil is retained.

- Many essential oils that are sold in the market are already diluted in carrier substances. It is important to check the labels of products if they contain 100% of the oil or only a trace amount as this would affect any preparations.

- Carrier oils or fixed oils are usually vegetable, seed or nut oils that have their own healing benefits. Combining these carriers with aromatic essential oils gives you combined health benefits.

- The best oils to use are those that are labeled organic and cold-pressed as they will also be absorbed by the body. Organic oils are grown without pesticides and insecticides, thereby making their oils even more potent, fresh, and safe.

Which Carrier Liquids Must Be Used?

A number of carrier oils and liquids are available in the market today. But here is a round-up of the most frequently used carrier oils today.

- The most popular oils to use as carriers include sweet almond oil and coconut oil. These are quite inexpensive, easy to find in stores and have light smells.

- Coconut oil is also an effective carrier substance. Pure coconut oil does have a distinct sweet nutty smell that some people can still detect even after mixing it with aromatic oils. Coconut oil mixed with your chosen aromatic oil can feel heavy, but it is suitable for use in people who have very dry skin and who need extra moisturizing properties.

- Sweet almond oil is ideal as a carrier for creating oil-based perfumes. Its sweet yet edible-smelling aroma is perfect for light day-to-day fragrance. It also has a lighter consistency than coconut oil and is absorbed by the skin quickly. Coconut oil tends to leave a greasy feeling.

- Grapeseed oil and sunflower seed oil are also good alternatives. They are commonly used in cosmetic preparations such as soaps, cleansers, deodorants, and lotions. These carrier oils are known to be highly moisturizing without clogging the pores.

- Some carrier oils also need to be used in conjunction with other carrier oils. While many swear by castor oil on its own, some skin types do react harshly to it and it can cause irritation and breakouts.

Essential Oils

- Jojoba, evening primrose and black cumin should also be kept at low proportions of at least a ratio of 2:10 with the rest of the solution. These oils are strongly potent and should be diluted accordingly to reap health benefits from them. Take note that black cumin oil is also called by other names including nutmeg flower, black caraway, black seed, Roman coriander and fennel flower.

- Balms or creams can also serve the purpose of carrier oils. They blend well with organic essential oils to create relaxing healthy concoctions that effortlessly slide on the skin. Balms and creams mixed with aromatic oils are great for a long, relaxing massage. The best to use are those that are also organic and natural like beeswax, Shea butter and coconut butter. Beeswax is best used mixed with other salves, but Shea butter and coconut butter are already good on their own.

- Pure distilled water can also be used as a carrier liquid. Water isn't as viscous as other carrier oils are, letting it reach more areas of the skin and body which oil-based carrier substances cannot do. Distilled water paired with a few drops of healing essential oils can cover areas that oils cannot enter like under nailbeds for the treatment of fungus.

    So, it is also a good idea to mix a few drops of essential oils into your bath water. However, it is essential that the water solution is agitated or shaken before use so that the oil can spread properly, as oil does not fully mix with water.

It is best to mix essential oils with carrier oils at the same time you use them. Do not mix them and store away the solution for later use. This not only affects the smells, but also the therapeutic effects of the essential oils.

Ingestion and Contraindications

Pointers to consider in essential oil ingestion, as well as contraindications to essential oil use, are presented below:

Most therapeutic essential oils are taken by the person externally (that is, through steaming, inhalation, massage, and oil bathing). Internal ingestion by swallowing the oils are often not advised. It may depend on what oil you're going to use, and what kind of ailment you want to eradicate using it.

It is possible to overdose on essential oils taken internally. There is really no evidence that ingesting essentials oils orally is more effective than inhalation or absorption through the skin. Though some oils are used in cooking and in preparations that may cause accidental swallowing (e.g., toothpaste, gargle), it is best to use them in small quantities and dilute in other edible and non-toxic substances.

Just because essential oils are natural, does not mean that they are not poisonous or harmful. They are highly concentrated and anything in high doses will have an adverse effect. Pure plant-sourced essential oils are very potent; one wrong preparation may cause more harm rather than the intended good.

Synthetic oils are composed of man-made chemicals that are very toxic and should not be used in any food or oral preparations. Nonetheless, pure essential oils are safe enough when used properly.

Who Should Not Take Essential Oil Therapies?

Essential oils should be kept out of reach of children. They can easily mistake them for drinks, especially when they are sweet-smelling and remind them of food. To be safe, invest in child-proof caps on the bottles or locks on cabinets and drawers where you store oils. Treat your essential oils as medicines so that your children will know that they should not be touched often.

Essential oils should always be diluted when being applied to the skin of infants and children. The tender skin of little ones is highly sensitive, and the potent essential oils might cause in minor burn injuries if essential oils are directly applied without diluting them.

When quite a large amount (i.e., more than a few drops) come in contact with a child's skin, liberally apply a light carrier oil like coconut, sweet almond or sunflower seed to sooth any possible irritation. Water will only spread the oil on the skin and increase the rate of absorption. Be sure to contact your health care practitioner for further steps in treating a child's affected skin.

Pregnant women should take caution when using essential oils. Though they have many benefits that can ease problems encountered by a woman during pregnancy, there are studies that show a correlation between the use of essential oils and changes in hormones and bodily functions. Many publications have lists of essential oils that are harmful to pregnant women and these include: sage, anise, myrtle, fennel, rosemary, cinnamon, basil, juniper berry, marjoram, nutmeg, clove, thyme, pimento berry, bay, valerian, hops, cistus, black pepper, cedar wood, myrrh, mace, peppermint, cumin, parsley seed, birch, wintergreen, wild tansy and calamus.

Use of essential oils during pregnancy could be harmful especially for moms suffering from elevated blood pressure levels. Essential oils may cause their blood pressures to arise even more, significantly cutting oxygen supply to their babies. The result is either preterm labor or a baby that's limp and weak upon birth. The baby might even require antibiotics because of a big risk in infection.

Although, effects do vary according to the individual. If using essential oils while pregnant, be mindful of sudden observable changes in the body like nausea, heart palpitations or headaches. Again, ingestion is not recommended and extra care should be taken when still breastfeeding.

Avoid UV radiation after applying essential oils on the skin, even when it has been diluted in carrier oils. This means minimizing exposure to the sun and artificial sources of UV rays. This is because ultraviolet light is absorbed at a faster rate by skin that has come in contact with essential oils. It can cause pigmentation and scarring.

In worse cases or in ultra-sensitive skin, it may even cause minor burn injuries. So, if you have to go out in the sun, wear both sunscreen and have physical protection like a UV protective umbrella or clothes with good coverage.

Adverse Reactions

A lot of people are allergic to even natural substances, and developing an allergic reaction to essential oils is possible. For example, a person with a known nut allergy (e.g., peanuts) should avoid all nut oils, especially because essential oils are concentrated versions of their plant sources. If unsure, it would be good to dilute an essential oil in a carrier oil and conduct a spot test on a small area of the skin. If no irritation develops in 24 hours, then the oil will be safe to use on the rest of the body.

It is also possible that the essential oil triggers a detoxification process in the body. While this is good, a sudden detoxifying effect can lead to physical effects similar to withdrawal symptoms (e.g., rashes, headaches, chills), so it will be good to introduce essential oils to the body in staggered amounts. If you still experience symptoms, lessen your exposure to the suspected oil trigger and gradually increase as your body gets used to it.

Oils to Avoid

These oils should never be used by amateur aromatherapists without professional knowledge of their chemical makeup:

Wormseed – This is a toxic oil derived from a perennial herb native to Eastern America. It can cause fatal kidney and liver poisoning. The oil contains *ascaridole,* an unstable compound that will explode when it comes into contact with heat or acids.

Wormwood – This is an oil coming from a perennial herb with pale yellow flowers. It has neurotoxic and narcotic properties. It is also an abortifacient oil, promoting menstruation even in the face of pregnancy. *Thujone* is its main substance contributing to its convulsant, neurotoxic properties.

Rue (when used on its own) – This oil comes from a native European shrub herbal plant. Its oil causes excessive sun sensitivity. It can be highly toxic to the skin and mucus membranes. It also causes abortion and brain toxicity.

Sassafras – This toxic oil is a carcinogenic, a cancer-inducing substance. The oil contains as much as 90% of the substance *safrole*, a lethal cancer-causing compound.

Savin – This oil has a bitter, repulsive taste and smells unpleasant. The Native American oil was once used to treat warts and blisters. But nowadays, it has been found to carry *podophyllotoxin*, a poisonous substance that can harm people even if used topically. Savin oil is also an abortifacient.

Tansy (distinct from wild tansy, which pregnant women should nonetheless avoid) – Tansy oil contains *thujone* substances and is yet another powerful abortifacient agent, making it highly unsuitable for pregnant women.

Southernwood – This is yet another abortifacient oil which stimulates a woman's uterus during pregnancy, causing miscarriages.

Horseradish – This plant oil is traditionally used to treat cough. However, it contains a substance called *allyl isothiocyanate* that is irritating to the mucus membranes, nasal passages, eyes, and skin.

Mugwort – Mugwort oil is extracted from an aromatic herb. However, it carries abortion-inducing properties and can become toxic to the brain cells.

Jaborandi leaf – Oils extracted from the jaborandi leaf may cause intensive sweating for as much as 9-15 ounces in a single dose alone. It's also a stomach irritant, inducing vomiting spiels and causing nausea.

Mustard – When mustard seeds are soaked in water, the oil of mustard is formed. This oil has a minimum of 90% *allyl isothiocyanate*, an irritant which affects the mucus membranes, eyes, nose, and skin.

Thuja – The oil from this plant is a poisonous abortion-inducing agent.

Pennyroyal – The plant oil can cause fatal damages to the liver and lungs. It also acts as a powerful abortifacient.

Yellow camphor (distinct from camphor) – Contains the toxic cancer-causing substance known as *safrole*. It can also cause vomiting, nausea, and convulsions.

Boldo leaf – This plant can induce convulsions of large proportions, even if consumed in a small amount.

Bitter almond (distinct from sweet almond) – Contains high amounts of the substance *cyanide*. This substance is obtained from the oil's prussic acid, and is widely known as a highly poisonous and lethal substance.

CHAPTER 6

Essential Oil Recipes

Are you now ready to try creating your very own DIY essential oil blends? There is a plethora of easy to create recipe blends for essential oil diffusion, steam inhalation, and massage. Read on and choose the recipe blends you think will be most beneficial to you. Try them out now and start living a naturally healthy life with the aid of aromatherapy essential oils!

For Diffusers

All these recipes are mixed with ¼ cup of water before pouring into your choice of diffuser, whether cold-air or warm. Always remember to use pure distilled water in your diffuser because tap water has impurities that don't only damage your unit but also adversely affect the potency of the essential oils you are mixing with it.

You can skip one or more of the essential oils in the recipe if you do not have them on hand. It is also possible to replace the missing essential oil with another oil you have in your collection that has similar properties.

Clean and Fresh Blend

This blend can make your house smell inviting and clean with a hint of citrus scents. It also deodorizes the air you inhale in any room you'd like it to be diffused. It is wonderful to have in the living room.

- 1 drop of lemon essential oil
- 1 drop of neroli essential oil

- 1 drop of grapefruit essential oil
- 2 drops of lavender essential oil
- 2 drops of rosemary essential oil

Air Freshener Blend

This blend can eliminate unwanted odors and freshen up the air. It is great to use in the bathroom or kitchen.

- 2 drops of lemon essential oil
- 1 drop of lime essential oil
- 1 drop of cilantro essential oil
- 1 drop of melaleuca essential oil
- 1 drop of lavender essential oil

Pick-Me-Up Blend

If you're in dire need of a fresh energizer, this citrusy-minty combo will surely delight you. This blend is best used in a cold-air diffuser and is great for bringing back mental sharpness and alertness. Diffuse this blend in times when you need a mood booster or a pick-me-upper.

- 2 drops of peppermint essential oil
- 2 drops of wild orange essential oil

Insect Repellant Blend

Bid *adieu* to those pesky insects with this blend! This recipe contains essential oils that insects do not like. These are effective on cockroaches, mosquitoes and flies. It is safe to use in a house with pets. It has been found that insects avoid these plants in the wild.

- 1 drop of citronella essential oil
- 1 drop of camphor essential oil
- 1 drop of eucalyptus essential oil
- 1 drop of basil essential oi
- 1 drop of thyme essential oil
- 1 drop of lemongrass essential oil

Spiced Chai Tea Blend

If you love chai tea, then you will enjoy this recipe. It is great as a pick-me-up in the morning or as an energy booster in the afternoon. Instead of plain distilled water, brew a half cup of chai tea. If using a cold-air diffuser, allow the tea to cool first. Do not attempt to steep a chai tea bag or loose leaves in your diffuser. Make the tea properly first in a separate pot or cup.

- 1 drop of ginger essential oil
- 1 drop of cinnamon bark essential oil
- 2 drops of clove essential oil
- 2 drops of cassia essential oil
- 2 drops of cardamom essential oil

Into the Woods Blend

This recipe has a nice woodsy feeling that will transport you in the middle of the woods. It is a bit heady, so only increase the number of drops of frankincense essential oil if you are used to heavier scents. Fans of light scents may find this too strong. For a more forest fresh scent, replace the frankincense with lemon or lime essential oil.

- 1 drop of cedar wood essential oil
- 1 drop of sandalwood
- 2 drops of white fir essential oil
- 3 drops of frankincense essential oil

Anti-Headache Blend

This blend is a great cure for headaches and you can diffuse this in your bedroom. You may substitute the eucalyptus essential oil with other mint oils like peppermint or spearmint that have all been found to alleviate headaches. You can also do a drop each of the three mint oils. The lavender and chamomile essential oils are calming will also help you sleep.

- 3 drops of eucalyptus essential oil
- 2 drops of lavender essential oil
- 1 drop of helichrysum essential oil
- 1 drop of chamomile essential oil
- 1 drop of rosemary essential oil

Insomnia Cure Blend

Try this recipe for an even deeper sleep than the one induced by the anti-headache blend. Too much vetiver essential oil can make you feel light-headed, so use less if you do not like that feeling. Some people even just dip a toothpick into the vetiver essential oil and use that to transfer a very small drop into the mixture instead of using a dropper.

- 2 drops of vetiver essential oil
- 2 drops of lavender essential oil
- 2 drops of chamomile essential oil

Garden Bloom Blend

Make your room smell like a flower garden in bloom with this recipe that consists of a blend of lovely flower essential oils.

- 2 drops of ylang ylang essential oil
- 2 drops of lavender essential oil
- 1 drop of rosemary essential oil
- 1 drop of geranium essential oil

Calming Blend

De-stress and calm your mind with this mystical blend that will remind you of crystal balls and magic shows. This scent is great for settling down for meditation.

- 1 drop of bergamot essential oil
- 1 drop of neroli essential oil
- 1 drop of patchouli essential oil
- 1 drop of sandalwood essential oil

Citrus Burst Blend

Long for the summer with this tropical recipe. This blend is also great for feeling better when you are sick or blue, especially in the winter months.

- 2 drops of lemon essential oil
- 1 drop of orange essential oil
- 1 drop of grapefruit essential oil
- 1 drop of lime essential oil

Sea Breeze Blend

Smell the ocean water and feel like you are on a vacation. Diffuse this blend in the bathroom as you take a bath to feel like you are relaxing on the beach.

- 3 drops of rosemary essential oil
- 2 drops of lavender essential oil
- 2 drops of bergamot essential oil
- 1 drop of eucalyptus essential oil

Take It Slow Blend

Are you giddy and anxious about something, but you want to calm down and just cannot find ways to relax? Use this blend especially before you sleep to help you relax, calm down, and shun out the jitters.

- 1 drop of ylang ylang essential oil
- 1 drop of bergamot essential oil
- 1 drop of patchouli essential oil

For Steaming

Time to bring out the large bowls and towels! These recipes are to be used in four cups of hot water poured into a bowl or pot.

Pore-cleansing Facial Steam

The steam opens up the pores so you can get into the deep-seated dirt on your skin. You can follow up this facial steam with a scrub and a splash of cold water to close the pores. This recipe is good for all skin types. You can also add dried flowers into the water like rose, sprigs of lavender and ylang ylang buds to intensify the scent.

Essential Oils

- 2 drops of chamomile essential oil
- 1 drop of rose otto essential oil
- 1 drop of lavender essential oil
- 1 drop of neroli essential oil1 drop of jasmine essential oil
- 1 drop of tea tree oil
- Dried flowers

Sinus-clearing Facial Steam

The method of steaming is perfect for clearing the sinuses and will benefit people suffering from clogged noses or allergic rhinitis. You can also add spearmint leaves into the water for that extra minty kick. Do not forget to close your eyes when steaming because the mint blend can make your eyes water.

- 7 drops of eucalyptus essential oil
- 4 drops of pine essential oil
- 3 drops of peppermint essential oil
- A sprig of torn spearmint leaves (optional)

Invigorating Facial Steam

This recipe stimulates the senses and makes for a good pick-me-up when you are sick or feeling cold. Add a stick of cinnamon bark while boiling the water for an extra spice.

- 3 drops of jasmine essential oil
- 2 drops of ylang ylang essential oil
- 2 drops of orange essential oil

- 2 drops of black pepper essential oil
- A stick of cinnamon (optional)

Mood Changing Facial Steam

Battle the blues and change your mood with this recipe. The scent will instantly make you feel more positive and will clear your head.

- 3 drops of bergamot essential oil
- 2 drops of basil essential oil
- 2 drops of lemon essential oil
- 2 drops of grapefruit essential oil
- 1 drop of ginger essential oil

Moon Facial Steam

This special recipe is for women who are on their period. It eases some menstrual symptoms and improves the mood.

- 4 drops of clary sage essential oil
- 2 drop of fennel essential oil
- 2 drops of rose geranium essential oil

For Massaging

These massage oils are safe to use on the skin and all over the body. However, do take note that facial skin reacts differently from the skin on other parts of the body, so if you have sensitive skin or acne-prone skin, use a light carrier oil like sunflower seed oil or grapeseed oil. You can also use these massage oils on the scalp and hair. For every recipe, add the essential oils to 15 mL of carrier oil of your choice. Review the previous chapter for the best carrier oil for you.

Muscle Relief Massage Oil

This recipe will feel warm on the skin because of the mint and cinnamon blend. It is wonderful to use after a workout.

- 4 drops of cinnamon essential oil
- 4 drops of eucalyptus essential oil
- 2 drops of ginger essential oil
- 1 drop of chamomile essential oil
- 1 drop of cajuput essential oil.

Refreshing Massage Oil

Get a massage with this oil after a long day's work. You will feel relaxed and ready to go to bed afterwards—or you might already fall asleep while getting massaged.

- 5 drops of spearmint essential oil
- 3 drops of basil essential oil
- 3 drops of rosemary essential oil
- 3 drops of bergamot essential oil
- 2 drops of lime essential oil

Achy Joints Massage Oil

This is good for individuals who are suffering from rheumatism. It soothes aching and painful joints without the need to resort to drugs.

- 8 drops of rosemary essential oil
- 8 drops of juniper berry essential oil
- 6 drops of lavender essential oil

Bath Massage Oil

Do this massage in the bath for very soft and supple skin. For easier application, you can mix this with organic bath salts or fine granulated brown sugar to create a bath scrub.

- 3 drops of fir essential oil
- 3 drops of spearmint essential oil
- 3 drops of geranium essential oil
- 3 drops of lemon essential oil
- 1 drop of juniper berry essential oil

Back Massage Oil

This massage oil is especially good to use on an aching back that is fatigued from slouching all day over a desk or a computer. The blend has an interesting herbal medicine smell that is highly therapeutic.

- 10 drops of lavender essential oil
- 5 drops of sandalwood essential oil
- 4 drops of rosemary essential oil
- 4 drops of geranium essential

Romantic Massage Oil

Have a romantic evening with your partner and enjoy the lovely scent of this massage oil blend. It is both spicy and sweet with a bit of a festive kick.

- 10 drops of ylang ylang essential oil
- 6 drops of sandalwood essential oil
- 3 drops of rose otto essential oil
- 3 drops of black pepper essential oil
- 3 drops of ginger essential oil
- 1 drop of nutmeg essential oil
- 1 drop of cinnamon essential oil

Immune Booster Massage Oil

Massage this all over your body to help strengthen your immune system. It is good to use during the flu season.

- 10 drops of tea tree essential oil
- 10 drops of geranium essential oil
- 8 drops of lemon essential oil
- 8 drops of thyme essential oil
- 5 drops of elemi essential oil
- 5 drops of myrrh essential oil

Detoxifying Massage Oil

Get rid of impurities in the body and feel much better after a massage with this oil blend.

- 4 drops of geranium essential oil
- 4 drops of rosemary essential oil
- 4 drops of juniper berry essential oil
- 4 drops of lavender essential oil
- 2 drops of tea tree essential oil

Conclusion

Thank you again for purchasing this book!

I hope this book was able to help you to become familiar with aromatherapy, its principles and practical applications.

The next step is to collect essential oils that are well-suited to your needs and incorporate them into your daily life and during healing. Just remember to treat your essential oils carefully. They are fragile yet strong and must be handled with proper care and caution. Go ahead and share what you have learned from this book with family and friends, so that they will have a wonderful life as well.

Finally, if you enjoyed this book, then I'd like to ask you for a favor, would you be kind enough to leave a review for this book on Amazon? It'd be greatly appreciated!

Thank you and good luck!

Printed in Great Britain
by Amazon